THE
LITTLE BOOK
of
ENERGY
MEDICINE

THE
LITTLE BOOK
of
ENERGY
MEDICINE

DONNA EDEN
with Dondi Dahlin

JEREMY P. TARCHER/PENGUIN
A member of Penguin Group (USA) Inc.
New York

JEREMY P. TARCHER/PENGUIN
Published by the Penguin Group
Penguin Group (USA) Inc., 375 Hudson Street, New York, New York 10014, USA ·
Penguin Group (Canada), 90 Eglinton Avenue East, Suite 700, Toronto, Ontario M4P 2Y3,
Canada (a division of Pearson Penguin Canada Inc.) · Penguin Books Ltd, 80 Strand,
London WC2R 0RL, England · Penguin Ireland, 25 St Stephen's Green, Dublin 2,
Ireland (a division of Penguin Books Ltd) · Penguin Group (Australia), 707 Collins Street,
Melbourne, Victoria 3008, Australia (a division of Pearson Australia Group Pty Ltd) ·
Penguin Books India Pvt Ltd, 11 Community Centre, Panchsheel Park, New Delhi–110 017, India ·
Penguin Group (NZ), 67 Apollo Drive, Rosedale, Auckland 0632, New Zealand
(a division of Pearson New Zealand Ltd) · Penguin Books, Rosebank Office Park,
181 Jan Smuts Avenue, Parktown North 2193, South Africa · Penguin China,
B7 Jaiming Center, 27 East Third Ring Road North, Chaoyang District, Beijing 100020, China

Penguin Books Ltd, Registered Offices: 80 Strand, London WC2R 0RL, England

Most Tarcher/Penguin books are available at special quantity discounts for
bulk purchase for sales promotions, premiums, fund-raising, and educational needs.
Special books or book excerpts also can be created to fit specific needs. For details, write
Penguin Group (USA) Inc. Special Markets, 375 Hudson Street, New York, NY 10014.

ISBN 978-1-58542-931-8

Cover design by Renne Rhae and Dondi Dahlin
Cover photograph by Christine Alicino
Cover model: Titanya Dahlin

Photographs by Rick Unis and Bernadette Unis-Johnston, www.narrativeimagesphoto.com

Printed in the United States of America
ScoutAutomatedPrintCode

BOOK DESIGN BY TANYA MAIBORODA

CONTENTS

The Five-Minute Daily Energy Routine

THE
LITTLE BOOK
of
ENERGY
MEDICINE

INTRODUCTION

You can be in greater control of your health right now! *The Little Book of Energy Medicine* is an easy and fun guide that is based on my thirty-four years of teaching people simple ways to enhance their energy and health. It is a book you can open daily to any page and find an exercise that helps you clear your mind and feel happier, more vital, and more alert.

What Exactly Is Energy Medicine and How Does It Work?

Nobel Prize–winning physicist Albert Einstein's formula $E = mc^2$ boils down to a simple concept: *energy is all there is*. There is *flowing* energy (what we usually simply think of as "energy") and *congealed* energy (matter). Everything in nature is one or the other—a mind-bending concept! Indeed, energy animates every cell and organ in your body. It is the Life Force and, put simply: when you have it, you are alive; when you don't, you aren't. Your body's relationship to this essential energy of nature has been evolving for millions of years. The energies that govern the way your body functions direct your immune system, hormones, and everything else that keeps you alive as decisively as a magnet will organize iron filings into distinct patterns. These energies have an amazing intelligence. They are much smarter than your intellect in keeping you healthy and in repairing you if you become ill. That said, you can mobilize your energies to keep your body and mind humming at their best. That is what Energy Medicine does. Energy Medicine is your body's best medicine.

In Energy Medicine, *energy* is the medicine and *energy* is also the patient. With energy as the *medicine*, the natural, vital, Life Force that is your birthright can be harnessed and directed to cure your ills and to uplift your spirit. With energy as the *patient*, you can restore energies that have become weak, disturbed, or out of balance and heal your body as well.

Flow, balance, and harmony can be noninvasively restored and maintained within your body's energy system by:

- Tapping, massaging, or holding specific energy points on the skin
- Tracing or swirling your hand above your skin along specific energy pathways
- Practicing exercises or postures designed to bring a feeling of calm and renewal
- Surrounding an area with healing energies

Just as there are different types of drugstore medicines, there are different types of Energy Medicine. Many can be traced back to ancient healing traditions such as yoga, qi gong, shiatsu, and acupuncture. Stone acupuncture needles that are eight thousand years old have been found in China. The body of a Neolithic man preserved in a frozen region between Austria and Italy had markings tattooed on his skin that correspond with the acupuncture points that would be used to treat the arthritis and stomach conditions revealed by a laboratory analysis of his body. Modern forms of Energy Medicine include Healing Touch, Therapeutic Touch, Touch for Health, Reiki, and Energy Kinesiology. The term "Energy Medicine" has been in use since the 1980s and more recently became a buzzword when referred to on both *The Oprah Winfrey Show* and *The Dr. Oz Show*.

Energy Medicine is both a complement to other approaches to medical care and a complete system for self-care and self-help. It can address physical illness and emotional or mental disorders, as well as promote high-level wellness and peak performance. Energies—both electromagnetic and more subtle energies—form the dynamic infrastructure of the physical body. The health of the body reflects the flow, balance, and harmony of those energies. When the body is not healthy, disturbances in its energies can be identified and treated.

The possibilities with Energy Medicine are, in fact, endless. With this *Little Book of Energy Medicine* you will:

* Learn a daily five-minute routine that keeps you feeling vibrant, alive, and full of energy
* Discover techniques for improving hormonal imbalances that cause hot flashes, sleep disturbance, or anxiety

- Access easy exercises to combat "everyday" ailments such as headaches and high blood pressure
- Practice energy techniques that counter psychological problems such as depression, mood swings, anger, and stress
- Be able to teach family, friends, and clients ways of maintaining and improving their own energy balance
- Learn to protect yourself from negative energies
- Support your body's immune system and ability to heal

What Are the Benefits of Energy Medicine?

- Do you wish you had more energy?
- Are you tired of taking pills for everyday aches and pains?
- Do you often wish there was a natural remedy when you aren't feeling well?
- Is your memory less sharp than it used to be?
- Do you find yourself dragging in the afternoon?
- Do you want to wake up more refreshed and eager for your day?

If your answer to any of these questions is "yes," then Energy Medicine is for you! Energy Medicine empowers you to be more in control of your body and your life. It doesn't cost anything to learn the Energy Medicine exercises in this book, and it is a gift you can give to yourself that keeps on giving.

Who Will Benefit from Energy Medicine?

- Anyone who wants to feel greater joy and vitality
- Ordinary people with no experience in healing themselves or healing others who are looking for answers to better health
- Doctors, nurses, massage therapists, acupuncturists, and others in health care who want to be more effective with their clients

Learning simple Energy Medicine exercises that will mobilize your energies instead of continuing to endure or medicate everyday pain and fatigue is a choice you can make right now. The pharmaceutical companies would like you to keep buying their drugs because they make billions of dollars from people who automatically reach for a bottle of pills to take their pain away. But doing this also taxes your liver, kidneys, and other organs when you could instead learn simple exercises that help heal your entire body, not just take away your aches and pains. Plus, Energy Medicine is safe. Medications are not necessarily safe, and in fact can interfere with your body's natural healing abilities. The U.S. Food and Drug Administration reports that accidental death from prescription drugs, even when they are taken correctly, is now the fourth leading cause of death in the United States. Additionally, when the FDA approves a medication for use by the general public, less than half of the serious drug reactions are known. *You become the guinea pig.*

Can Anyone Use Energy Medicine?

The good news is, "Yes!" Anyone can learn and use Energy Medicine! From this guide, you will have practical and straightforward techniques that you can use immediately. Energy Medicine is the safest, most organic, most accessible, and most affordable medicine there is. Energy Medicine teaches you how to participate more fully and knowledgeably in your own healing, health, and well-being. No devices are necessary. You will use the touch of your hands and your own energies to lift your spirits and foster a healthier, happier life. You can start right now by trying one of the exercises in these pages. There is no reason to wait. Try one now and start feeling better today—and every day, for the rest of your life.

What Energy Medicine Is and Is Not

"Diagnosis" and "treatment" within Energy Medicine have different meanings than they have within traditional medicine. The focus is not on symptoms or illness; the focus is on keeping the body's *energy system* strong, vital, harmonious, and healthy. In Energy Medicine, you "diagnose" or assess the energy system, not the illness. Symptoms provide clues about where the energy system needs attention. Likewise, treatment is not the treatment of symptoms or illness; it is the treatment of the energy system.

These distinctions are vital not only because it is legal to educate people to keep their body's energies healthy but not legal for unlicensed people to diagnose and treat illness. They are also vital because they demonstrate a fundamentally different way of thinking about health and illness that directs your attention to the energetic foundation of staying healthy. The techniques suggested here may be used along with traditional medical treatments. They will generally complement them, and your health care professional will probably be interested to know what other interventions you are using.

How Do I Get Started?

You don't need any special tools to get started with Energy Medicine. All you need is the desire to be healthy. Many people spend their adulthood feeling tired most of the time. This book will help you feel energized and boost your immune system so headaches, high blood pressure, coughs, colds, and flu don't run you down every year.

Preventive medicine is crucial in a day and age of rising medical costs and many people left without health insurance. Luckily, preventive medicine is fairly easy to begin. It only takes a decision to start the exercises in this book and perform them daily.

How to Use This Book

This book is a user-friendly guide. You can pick it up and read the instructions in any order. It is designed for people who are ready to try Energy Medicine for the first time and want a quick and easy way to get started, or if you have already used Energy Medicine in the past and want a simple guide to keep with you for easy reference. You do not need any special background or training to be able to get health benefits from the exercises presented here. They are ready for you to use now, and you will probably find that you receive benefits almost immediately. Depending on your personal strengths and challenges, some of the exercises are likely to work better for you than others. If you are interested in deeper study or would like more instruction and explanation about a certain technique, you will want to pick up my more comprehensive books, *Energy Medicine* and *Energy Medicine for Women*.

Meridians, Acupressure Points, Chakras, and the Aura

Meridians: The fourteen meridians are the body's main energy pathways. In the way an artery transports blood, a meridian transports energy. The meridians carry a flow of energy that adjusts metabolism, and vitalizes every organ and every physiological system in the body. These meridian pathways bring energy

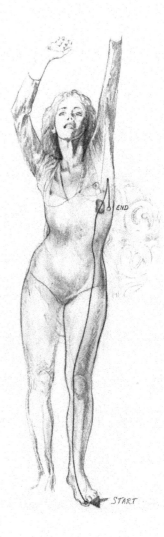

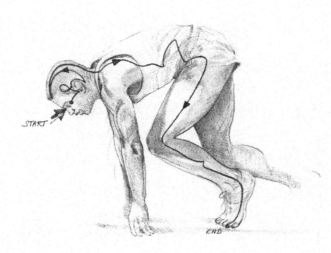

Spleen and gallbladder meridians, shown here, are two of the body's 14 meridian pathways.

to the immune, nervous, endocrine, circulatory, respiratory, digestive, skeletal, muscular, and lymphatic systems. These pathways exist within the "subtle body"—the invisible field that surrounds and permeates the physical body. Medical students don't find these subtle energies when they dissect cadavers.

Our ancient ancestors needed to sense the energies of plants to know if they were nutritious or poisonous; to be able to feel the energies of an approaching predator; and to know when the energies of their children or mate were out of harmony so they could keep those they depended upon healthy and focused. These abilities helped them survive. Teachings and traditions for balancing the body's energies to keep people vital can be found in most ancient civilizations. The Chinese were probably the first to write down a system for working with the body's energies, focusing on the acupuncture meridians, and acupuncture is still healing people today. Meanwhile, contemporary scientists are finding ways to demonstrate and measure subtle energies and energy fields.

Acupressure Points: Acupressure is a safe and holistic healing art that was developed in China over five thousand years ago. This ancient technique uses the fingers to press key points along the meridian lines on the body where the energy pools. Acupressure has been effective in the relief of trauma, emotional pain, and physical pain, as well as boosting the immune system, beauty treatments, better sex, back care, relaxation, combatting addictions, and much more. Acupuncture and acupressure use the same points and meridians, but acupuncture employs needles while acupressure uses the fingers.

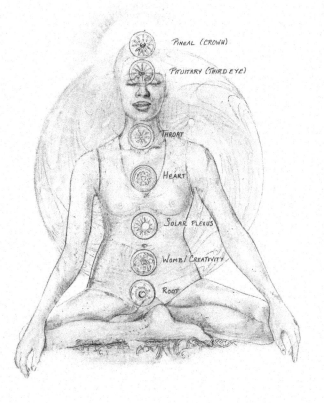

PINEAL (CROWN)

PITUITARY (THIRD EYE)

THROAT

HEART

SOLAR PLEXUS

WOMB / CREATIVITY

ROOT

Chakras: The chakras are concentrated centers of energy located up the midline of the body from the base of the spine to the top of the head. There are seven chakras, which are believed to energetically record every emotionally significant event you experience. Trained practitioners can work with the chakras by holding their hands over the chakra and moving the energy.

The Aura: The aura is a field that surrounds your entire body with an energetic embrace. Scientists who have detected the aura's energy call it the "biofield." It is a multilayered protective sphere of energy that interacts with the energies within you as well as with the atmosphere around you. Your aura is made up of many ever-changing colors that some practitioners are able to see, interpret, and adjust.

ENERGY
EXERCISES

for

COMMON
AILMENTS

Arm Attachment Stress Points

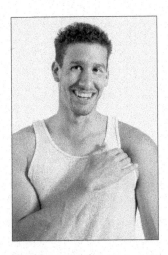

Find the area where your arm meets your body. Push your fingers in with pressure, massaging the length of the arm-body connection. Breathe out through your mouth whenever you feel any tenderness.

- Stimulates the lymphatic system, which helps move toxins out of the body
- Increases production of white blood cells, strengthening your immune system
- Helps your body remove toxins
- Strengthens your body and aura
- Calms emotions

How it works: The circulatory system and the lymphatic system are the two systems that send fluid throughout your body. Your heart pumps blood for your circulatory system, but your lymphatic system does not have a pump. Its fluids are pumped by movement—walking, running, exercising. But with our sedentary lifestyles, the lymphatic system—which is responsible for removing physical toxins and stale energies—gets clogged. Massaging the reflex points at the arm-body junction gets your lymph flowing so it can remove toxins.

The Celtic Weave

The Celtic weave "weaves" your aura and builds its protective surrounding. It organically connects all of the energy systems of your body together.

- Strengthens the energy field around you (your "aura")
- Protects you from harmful energies in the environment

How it works: Your aura protects you from the effects of energy pollutants in the atmosphere such as those caused by high-voltage wires and fluorescent lights, as well as the vibrations of people who are stressed, angry, or depressed. Celtic weaving laces your aura with all of your other energetic systems and helps hold your entire energetic structure together. You are literally making figure eights with both arms from the top of your body to the bottom. When the Celtic weave is dynamically engaged, you have a sense of power, a feeling of being charged, and your energies really start humming.

▼

Rub hands together, shake them off, face palms, and try to feel the energy between them. Rub and shake again, place palms close to ears, and take a deep breath.

Inhale and bring your elbows together. Exhale, cross your arms and swing out. This motion should make a figure eight with both arms, not just a crossing of the arms. Cross and swing them out again in a figure-eight motion.

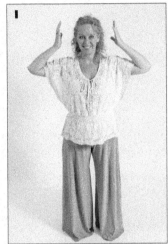

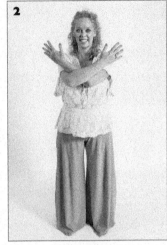

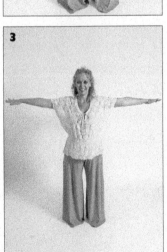

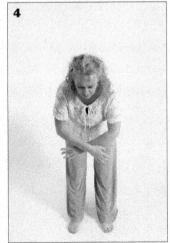

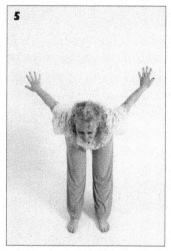

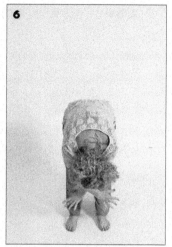

Bend forward, repeat, and cross arms over upper legs. Swing out again, in front of ankles. Bend knees, turn palms forward, scoop up energy, stand, and pour that energy all over your body.

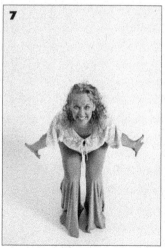

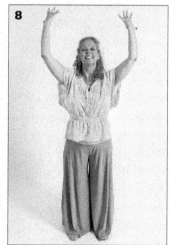

Connecting Heaven and Earth

A wonderfully energizing exercise that releases energy stuck in your joints and allows you to feel refreshed. Can be used alone or as a part of the Five-Minute Daily Energy Routine.

- Releases energy, including energies picked up from other people and toxic environments
- Brings fresh oxygen to the cells, which activates endorphins and supports feelings of joy
- Activates the immune system
- Helps ease insomnia

How it works: Connecting Heaven and Earth is one of the most popular exercises in Energy Medicine because it makes people feel so good. It opens the meridians and brings many people a feeling of joy and happiness. This powerful stretch for the hips, waist, and torso is one of my favorite ways to quickly renew myself if I'm feeling sluggish.

▼

1 *Start with your hands on your thighs, with your fingers spread.*

2 *Inhale through your nose, bring your arms out and together in a prayer position. Exhale through your mouth.*

3 *Inhaling through your nose, stretch one arm up and one arm down, pushing with your palms. Hold, exhale through your mouth, and return to the prayer position. Switch arms and repeat.*

4 *Drop your arms down, fold your body forward at the waist, and relax with your knees slightly bent. Take two breaths before slowly returning to a standing position.*

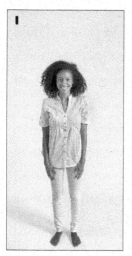
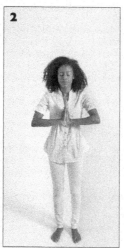
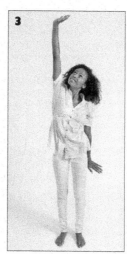
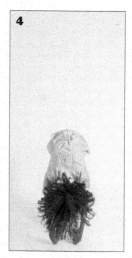

Cook's Hookup

Variation of the Wayne Cook Posture. Useful as a shortcut for someone who cannot get into the full Wayne Cook Posture.

* Focuses the mind
* Enhances learning capacity
* Brings out your best in a performance or confrontation

How it works: This procedure is a modification of the Wayne Cook Posture (page 56). It is named to honor Wayne Cook, a pioneer in the field of bioenergetic force fields. Perhaps more than any other single approach that I teach, the Wayne Cook Posture can calm you, and help you better understand and confront the problems that you face. It is very effective when you are so upset that you find yourself yelling, crying, or sinking into despair. You will usually begin to feel less overwhelmed almost immediately. Holding the ending pose (#3) with an affirmation of how well you will do in your performance or encounter will turbocharge your affirmation.

▼

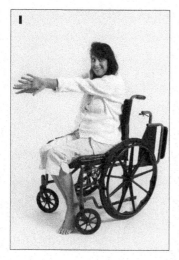

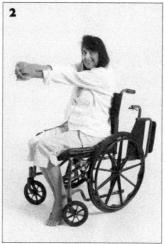

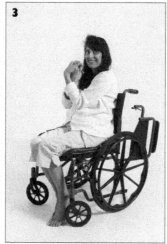

1. *Extend your left hand in front of you, turn your palm to the side, and cross your right hand over your wrist.*

2. *Clasp your fingers together and pull your hands underneath and up to your chest. If you are sitting, cross your ankles.*

3. *Take four slow, deep breaths, in through your nose and out through your mouth.*

Crown Pull

The Crown Pull can be done as part of the Five-Minute Daily Energy Routine or simply when you are congested in your head or mind.

* Stimulates blood flow to your head
* Strengthens memory
* Opens the crown chakra, which is associated with spirituality and inspiration
* Helps overcome insomnia
* Can help alleviate headaches

How it works: Stress causes energy to accumulate and stagnate at the top of your head. The Crown Pull releases this energy. It can clear the cobwebs from your mind and bring calm to your nervous system. It can also often take away a headache or stress-induced stomachache. Over the years, I've had many people tell me they use it as a prelude to meditation or other spiritual practices.

▼

1 Apply pressure to forehead and slowly pull your fingers apart stretching the skin. Breathe deeply, in through your nose and out through your mouth. Next, place your fingertips on the top of your head and repeat the stretch.

2 Repeat this pattern starting at the top, center, and back of your head. Continue until you reach the base of your neck.

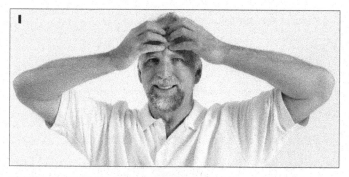

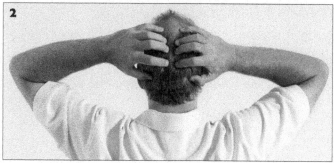

Expelling the Venom

When you are feeling angry or frustrated or you want to find the righteous anger within you, this is a good exercise to do.

- Moves rage out of your body
- Frees congested energies
- Unblocks the spirit

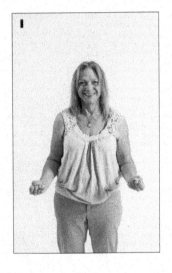

Stand up straight. Put your arms out in front of you, bend your elbows slightly, make fists with the insides of your wrists facing up, and take a very full breath. Swing your arms behind you and up over your head. Hold here for a moment. Reach way up, turn your fists so your fisted fingers are facing each other, and rush your arms down the front of your body as you emphatically release your fists. Let out your breath and your emotions with a *whooosh* sound or any other powerful sounds that come naturally. Repeat several times. This will probably feel good. The last time, bring your arms down in a slow and controlled manner, blowing your breath out of your mouth as you go.

How it works: This exercise evokes and releases the energies of anger, upset, and frustration. It is a primal and effective way to let go of stress and anger. Becoming more viscerally familiar with anger makes space for healthy assertiveness.

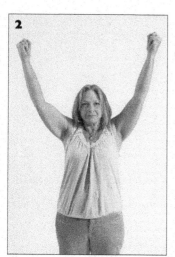

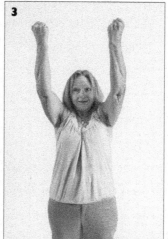

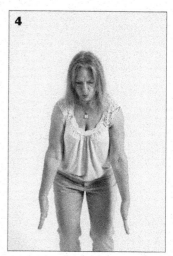

Fear Tap

The Fear Tap can be done any time you are feeling anxious or scared. It can also alter the underlying pattern of a long-standing phobia. Tapping energy points traces back to a five-thousand-year-old healing tradition and is a friendly, nonintrusive way to instantly shift the brain's electrochemistry.

- Calms the Triple Warmer meridian, which governs the flight-or-flight response
- Reduces irrational fear
- Soothes the body
- Steadies the mind

Locate the area on the back side of your hand, halfway between your wrist and fingers, between your ring finger and "pinkie" finger. Tap this area with two or three fingers of your other hand for 30 to 60 seconds, breathing in through your nose and out through your mouth. Switch hands. Another option is to place one hand over your heart and tap on the hand as instructed above.

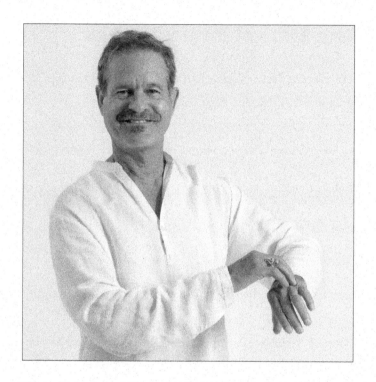

How it works: Being afraid might be about something specific, but fear is also sometimes irrational and generalized. It can create stress, agitation, and exhaustion. Tapping on these acupressure points can shift energies of fear and gently alleviate unwanted thoughts in a matter of minutes.

The Four Memory Pumps

This exercise restores long-term and short-term memory for most people. It also feels great!

* Enhances the flow of cerebrospinal fluid, which helps us think more clearly
* Improves memory

Sit or stand comfortably. Rub all over your head with your knuckles or fingers to open the energies in your head. Take a deep breath, in through the nose and out through the mouth.

How it works: Oxygen-rich cerebrospinal fluid is drawn up the spine, supporting the nervous system and delivering nutrients to the brain. This fluid protects the brain and spinal cord from trauma brought about by movement, falls, and blows.

1   *Place the palm of your left hand on the left side of your head with your fingers crossing over the top of your head. Your right hand goes on the middle of your chest. Take three deep breaths.*

2   *Keeping your right hand on your chest, move your left hand so that your palm is on your forehead and your fingers are stretched over the top of your head. Take three deep breaths.*

3   *Move your left hand to your chest, your right hand to the right side of your head (as in photo 1, but with your left and right hands reversed) and take three deep breaths.*

4   *Keep your left hand at your chest, place the palm of your right hand on the back of your head, and hold for three breaths.*

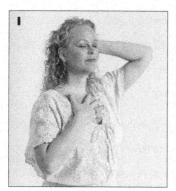
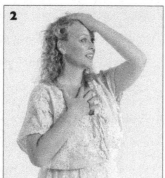
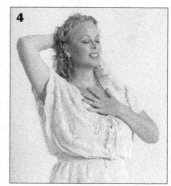

The Four Thumps

By thumping four specific sets of points on your body, a technique I call the "Four Thumps," you can activate a sequence of responses that will restore you. The Four Thumps are a part of the Five-Minute Daily Energy Routine.

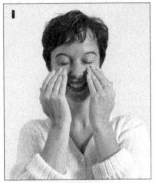

- Boosts your immune system
- Balances blood chemistry and electrolytes
- Helps with the metabolism of food
- Reduces toxins and stress
- Promotes clear thinking

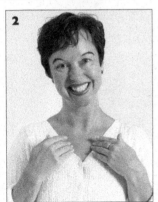

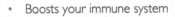

1 *Place the pads of your fingers beneath your cheekbones, next to your nose. Thump firmly for 15 seconds. This helps to drain sinuses and clear the lymph glands in the neck. It can also release tension and reduce excessive worry.*

2 *To locate these points, place your forefingers on your collarbone and move them inward toward the U-shaped notch at the top of your breastbone (about where a man would tie his tie). Move*

your fingers to the bottom of the U. Then go to the left and right about an inch and thump firmly for 10 to 15 seconds.

3 Place the fingers of either or both hands in the center of your sternum, at the thymus gland. Thump firmly for about 10 to 15 seconds.

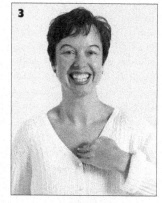

4 Thump the neurolymphatic spleen points firmly for 10 to 15 seconds with your fingers or knuckles. They are beneath the breasts and down one rib.

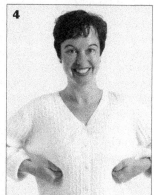

How it works: Certain points on your body, when tapped with your fingers, will impact your energy field in predictable ways, sending electrochemical impulses to your brain and releasing neurotransmitters. These are four such that work in combination to "charge your batteries." Please use a very firm tap or "thump." If there is any tenderness, that usually means this exercise is good for you and can help release toxins in clogged areas.

Gait Reflexes

On top of your feet, in the spaces between the bones that correspond with the spaces between the toes, are your gait reflexes: acupressure points between the metatarsal bones. Fatigue may be caused by a disturbance in your walking gait or just from being on your feet a lot. This means that the normal coordination of the muscles used in walking becomes tiring. Massaging the gait reflexes can help to restore your energy.

- Helps to "ground" you
- Releases tension and is wonderfully relaxing
- Frees energy that tends to become clogged in your feet

With your fingers below each foot and your thumbs on the gait reflex, massage the energy down each of the five gait reflexes with your thumbs. Pull the energy off your toes. Spread the thumbs with pressure to the outside of the feet.

How it works: The gait reflexes are acupressure points in the feet and linked to a variety of muscles that function during walking. These include muscles in the shoulders and hips. Massaging your gait reflexes boosts energy.

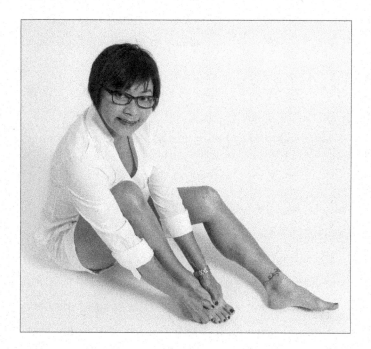

Heaven Rushing In

This exercise can connect you to the larger forces of the universe and your spirituality.

- When you don't know what else to do, this practice initiates healing
- Brings comfort and opens your intuition when you are feeling lonely or in despair
- Allows you to direct healing energies to specific areas of your body

How it works: In the middle of the chest, near the heart, is a vortex called "Heaven Rushing In." Powerful healing energies can be directed into this vortex. When you perform this exercise and sense the healing energies, it reminds you that you are not alone in this universe. Notice the insights that may come to you. If you need healing in a specific spot, take the energy that has streamed into your heart chakra and, with your hands, bring it to an area of your body that needs healing. For instance, if you have hip pain, you can end this exercise by placing your hands on your hips.

1   *Stand tall and ground yourself with your hands on your thighs. Breathe in through your nose and out through your mouth throughout the exercise.*

2   *Reach out and up and bring your hands together in a prayer position.*

3   *Touch the heavens with both hands by raising your arms and opening your hands. Look up. Know that you are not alone. Unlimited energies and healing forces are there to meet you whenever you ask.*

4   *Scoop up the healing energy and place it on your heart chakra in the middle of your chest.*

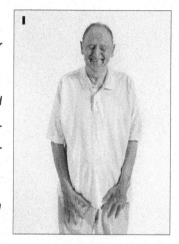

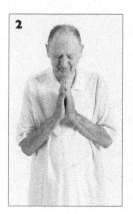

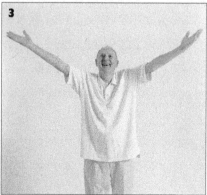

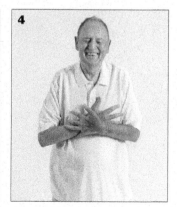

Holding Another's Stress Points

You can hold these points yourself or you can have a friend hold them so you can fully relax into the experience of feeling your worries melt away.

- Helps when feeling upset or if you have the "blues"
- Releases tension
- Helps you think more clearly

How it works: When you are stressed, blood leaves your forebrain and goes into your trunk and limbs to support the fight-or-flight response. Without enough blood in your forebrain, it is hard to think clearly or handle stress. When you hold the neuro-vascular points, the electromagnetic energy in your fingers draws the blood back into your forebrain. You are lifted out of stress.

Sit comfortably and have your partner place the palm of one hand on the forehead, the other on the back of the head. Breathe slowly and deeply, in the nose and out through the mouth. Partner can hold for 3 to 4 minutes.

ALTERNATIVE: Have your partner place fingertips on your forehead, touching the area above the eyes, and wrap hands around the temples.

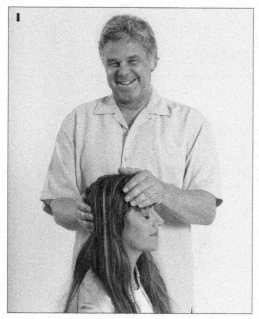

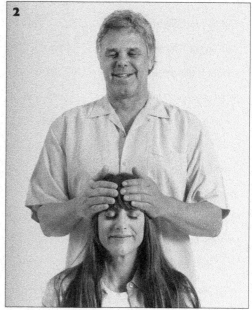

Holding Your Own Stress Points (Neurovasculars)

Holding the neurovasculars (the two areas on your forehead, located about an inch above each eye) helps when blood leaves the forebrain. This happens in many situations, including during hot flashes for women in menopause.

1 Lightly place your finger-tips on your forehead, covering the frontal eminences (the bumps on your forehead directly above your eyes). Put your thumbs on your temples next to your eyes, breathing deeply. As the blood returns to your forebrain over the next few minutes, you will find yourself beginning to think more clearly. It is that simple!

- Prevents blood from leaving the forebrain
- Calms the part of your brain that initiates the fight-or-flight response
- Assists in repatterning unwanted habits

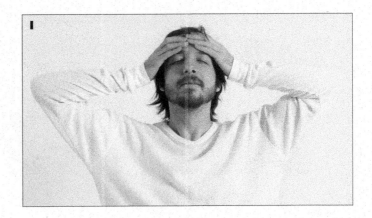

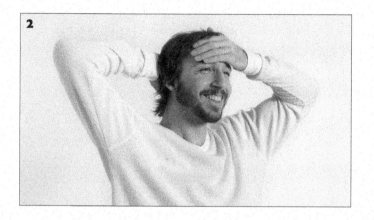

2

How it works: When a stress sends you into the fight-or-flight response, up to 80 percent of the blood leaves your forebrain to go into your arms and chest to fight, or into your legs to run. A simple technique of placing the pads of your fingers on your forehead and your thumbs on your temples impacts circulation and brings blood back to your head. The points on your forehead are called "neurovasculars," and lightly holding them can shift you out of the stress response. You can also use this exercise to diffuse a traumatic memory.

2 *Lay one palm on your forehead and the other on the back of your head. Hold them there for 2 to 3 minutes, breathing deeply and comfortably. Holding the front neurovascular points returns blood to your forebrain and balances the circulation of blood throughout your body. Holding your other hand behind your head sedates the fear points and calms your hypothalamus.*

Homolateral/Cross-Crawl Repatterning

This repatterning exercise supports the crossover patterns in your body's energies that are necessary for coordination, healing, and vitality. Can be used alone or as part of the Five-Minute Daily Energy Routine.

- Helps you think more clearly and improves coordination
- Speeds the healing process
- Facilitates the crossover of energy between the brain's right and left hemispheres
- Gives you more energy and can lift you out of depression or fuzzy thinking

How it works: You may feel tired during this exercise, but it will leave you feeling reenergized. Homolateral repatterning helps to reset the nervous system and supports the flow of information between the two hemispheres of the brain.

1   *Homolateral March: While standing, lift your left arm and left leg simultaneously. As you let them down, raise your right arm and right leg. Repeat several times.*

2   *Cross-Crawl: Lift your left arm and right leg simultaneously. As you let them down, raise your right arm and left leg. Repeat several times.*

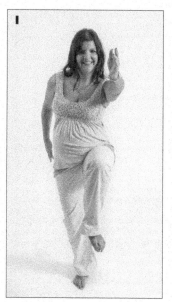 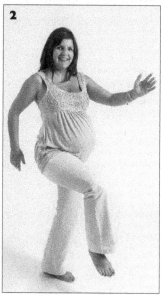

TIPS ON HOW TO DO IT:

Begin this sequence with the Homolateral March (same leg, same arm). Repeat the march 4 to 5 times before switching to the Cross-Crawl (opposite leg, opposite arm). Repeat the Cross-Crawl 4 to 5 times. Go back and forth between the Homolateral March and the Cross-Crawl several times until you feel that they are easy and comfortable to do. There should also be a feeling of being reenergized. Always end the sequence with the Cross-Crawl. Reminder: the Homolateral March and Cross-Crawl are essentially exaggerated walks.

Hookup

The Hookup can be done at the end of the Five-Minute Daily Energy Routine or simply when you are feeling a bit "off."

- Creates a connection between your central meridian (which sends energy up the front of your body) and the governing meridian (which sends energy up your spine)
- Increases your coordination
- Reduces anxiety
- Strengthens your aura

Place one hand with your middle finger in your navel and the other hand with your middle finger in your "third eye" (between your eyebrows). Push in and pull up.

How it works: The Hookup is one of the most powerful tools I know to quickly get yourself feeling better physically and

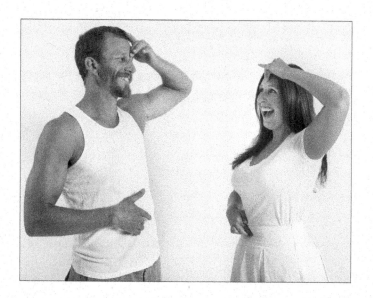

emotionally. The Hookup supports the nervous system and has been known to stop seizures. During the Hookup, breathe deeply and slowly in through your nose and out through your mouth 5 or 6 times. You can close your eyes or leave them open. Always find the way that feels right for you! That's how your body's energies talk to you.

Hooking Up a Friend

The "Hookup" is the best single technique for keeping the aura solid. It is wonderful for comforting a baby or toddler.

- Helps overcome insomnia
- Stabilizes your entire energy system
- Increases coordination

Have your friend sit or lie down and place the middle finger of one hand on the third eye (between the eyebrows above the bridge of the nose) and the middle finger of your other hand in the navel. Gently press each finger into the skin, pull it upward, and hold for 15 to 30 seconds.

How it works: The Hookup connects the central and governing meridians, bridging their energies between the front and back of your body and between your head and torso. It is one of my most used techniques for quickly centering myself. It has immediate neurological consequences, including stopping seizures.

TO COMFORT A BABY OR TODDLER: Place your left hand under the baby's neck and head, and let the baby's head rest there. Place your other hand on the baby's stomach, below the belly button. Babies are usually very responsive to the energies that will flow between your hands.

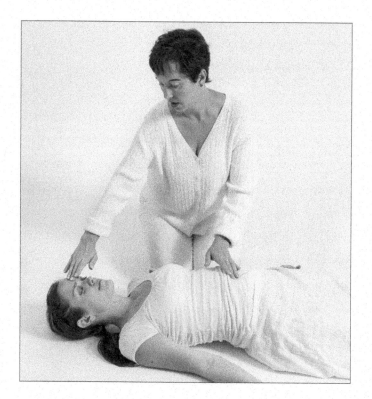

Spinal Flush

This is a kind gift to give a friend who is feeling run down or upset. This exercise is part of the Five-Minute Daily Energy Routine.

- Energizes your body
- Removes toxins from lymphatic system
- Clears stagnant energy

Lean into a chair or wall, or lie facedown. Partner should deeply massage on either side of the spine, from the base of the neck to the bottom of the sacrum. The thumbs are used to apply deep pressure in a circular motion for about 5 seconds on each point. Once at the bottom of the sacrum, your partner can repeat the spinal flush or "sweep" the energies off the body. From the shoulders, and with an open hand, your partner sweeps all the way down the back, down the legs, and off the feet 2 or 3 times.

How it works: The Spinal Flush works with your lymphatic system. The lymph has no pump of its own, but you pump it whenever you move your body. You can also pump it by massaging your neurolymphatic reflex points. Congested neurolymphatic reflex points feel sore when massaged. For this reason, they are not hard to locate. And, there are so many of these points so close to one another that you won't miss them. Lymph plays a key role in your immune system by helping fight conditions ranging from colds to cancer.

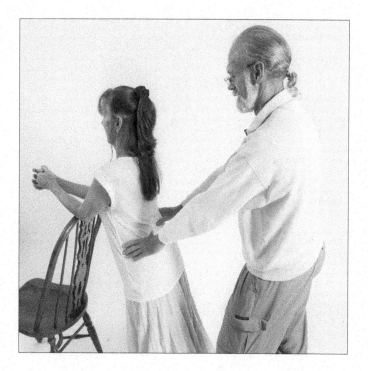

NOTE: *If you are alone, this exercise can also be achieved by using tennis balls, or any ball that is comfortable under your back. Lie on your back and place the tennis balls under either side of your spine, gently rocking your body so the tennis balls deeply massage the lymphatic points. This takes some practice but many people say they can achieve a very good lymphatic massage by working the tennis balls down the spine from the neck to the bottom of the sacrum.*

Taking Down the Flame

This exercise could have easily been named "Taking Down the Hyperactivity." If you do this with a child, it will usually help keep them more focused and will calm you as well.

- Calms you when you feel out of control
- Reduces panic
- Helps ground you
- Can lower blood pressure

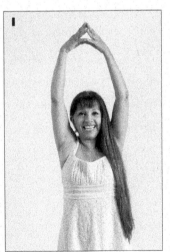 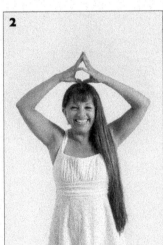 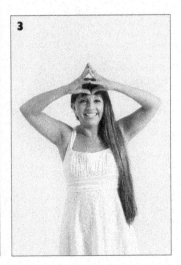

Stand with your hands on your thighs, fingers spread. Breathe in deeply through your nose and out through your mouth. Swing your arms out, bringing them over your head until the fingertips and thumbs of each hand meet.

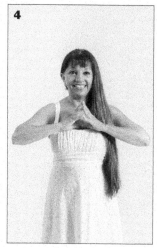

Exhaling, lower your thumbs to the top of your head. Hold and inhale deeply. Exhale and place your thumbs between your eyebrows. Hold and inhale deeply. Exhale and place your thumbs on your thymus point, between your breasts. Hold and inhale deeply.

As you let your breath out, take your thumbs down to your navel and "triangle" your fingers below your navel and flatten your hands. Breathe in deeply, smooth your hands down the front of your legs while bending forward at the waist, and let them hang.

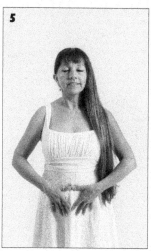

Breathe in deeply and slowly stand, placing one vertebra on top of the other. Lift your shoulders toward your ears and drop them.

How it works: Taking Down the Flame connects all the chakras for a "quickie" chakra balancing. Additionally, it literally "takes down the flame"—panic or anxiety you may be feeling. It grounds you and makes you feel calm and at peace again, allowing you to handle whatever problems you have.

Tapping In the Joy

You can literally tap joy into your nervous system so it begins to create a pattern of happiness in your life.

- Increases your joy
- Helps you imprint the good moments in your life into your nervous system
- Shifts your mind to move toward the positive

The next time you are feeling happy, or experiencing a wave of gratitude, awe, or appreciation, tap it in at your third eye. Tap with the middle finger of either hand, between the eyebrows, above the bridge of your nose for 5 to 10 seconds. This sends the positive feeling into your energy field through the first acupressure point on your nervous system.

How it works: Tapping at your "third eye" while remembering good moments in your life, recalling something that made you laugh, or giving an affirmation of gratitude for your body, your mind, your life, or another person is powerful Energy Medicine.

It creates a rhythmic pulse of positive energy. This is the first acupressure point on the bladder meridian, which helps govern the central nervous system. It is also known in yoga tradition as the "third eye." It is associated with intuition and psychic awareness. Tapping on the "third eye" point while you feel joy pulses the joy throughout your nervous system. It also trains your nervous system to be more joyful.

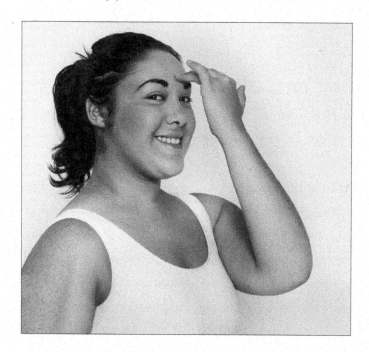

Triple Warmer Smoothie

The "smoothie" calms the Triple Warmer meridian, which runs from the fourth finger, up the outside of the arm, behind the ear, and to the outside of the eyes. It governs the immune system, the emergency response to threat (fight, flight, or freeze), and the ability to form physiological and behavioral habits for managing stress or threat.

- Reduces fear and anxiety
- Releases tension
- Helps overcome insomnia
- Helps with body temperature and hot flashes

Place the pads of your fingers on your temples. Take a deep breath in through your nose and out through your mouth. On another deep in-breath, slowly slide your fingers up and over your ears, maintaining some pressure. On the out-breath, take them around and behind your ears, down your neck, and hang your fingers on your shoulders. When you are ready, push your fingers into your shoulders, drag them across the front of your shoulders, and let them go.

How it works: The Triple Warmer meridian is a little different from the other meridians because it is not represented by a physical organ. Instead, it is defined by its function. Its purpose is to enlist energies from other meridians to better respond to stress. It truly is a "human thermostat" that governs the endocrine system, the autonomic nervous system, basic drives, and appetite balance. Blockage in the triple warmer meridian can manifest itself in many ways, including a stiff neck, water retention, shock, and emotional sensitivity. The Triple Warmer Smoothie sedates the triple warmer meridian and helps to restore peace and calm.

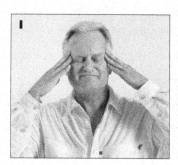
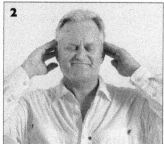
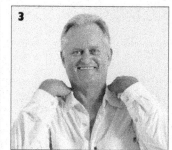

Wayne Cook Posture

The Wayne Cook Posture can be done when you are feeling overwhelmed or confused. It is also part of the Five-Minute Daily Energy Routine.

- Takes you out of stress and feeling overwhelmed
- Helps you think more clearly
- Helps you to process and retain information
- Brings out your best in a performance or confrontation

How it works: This technique is effective even when the upset is so intense that you are unable to quit crying, are finding yourself snapping or yelling at others, are sinking into despair, or are feeling that you are beyond exhaustion. It helps process stress hormones, and almost immediately you will begin to feel less crazy and less overwhelmed. This procedure is named to honor Wayne Cook, a pioneering researcher of bioenergetic force fields, who invented the approach that I have modified into the form presented here.

1. Place your right foot over your left knee. Wrap your left hand around your right ankle and your right hand around the ball of your right foot. Breathe in slowly through your nose and out through your mouth. Repeat this 4 to 5 times. Switch to the other foot. Place your left foot over your right knee. Wrap your right hand around your left ankle and your left hand around the ball of your left foot. Use the same breathing.

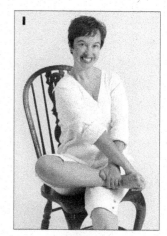

2. Uncross your legs and place your fingertips together forming a pyramid. Bring your thumbs to rest on your "third eye," just above the bridge of your nose. Breathe slowly in through your nose. Then breathe out through your mouth, repeating 4 or 5 times. Finally, allow your thumbs to separate slowly across your forehead, pulling the skin. Allow your hands to simply drop into your lap.

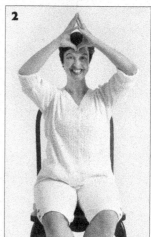

Zip-up

The Zip-up creates a natural form of self-protection from toxins and negative energy in the environment. This can be done alone or as a part of the Five-Minute Daily Energy Routine.

- Protects you from absorbing negative energies and environmental toxins
- Lifts your energy and spirit
- Can be used with affirmations and positive imagery

How it works: When you are feeling sad or vulnerable, the central meridian, one of the two energy pathways that govern your central nervous system, can be like a radio receiver that channels other people's negative thoughts and energies into you. It's as if you are open and exposed. Pulling our hands up the central meridian draws energy along the meridian line and "zips it up," which will help you feel more confident and positive about yourself. You can zip up the central meridian as often as you wish. By tracing it in this manner, you strengthen the meridian, and the meridian strengthens you.

1 Briskly tap the K-27 points to assure that your meridians are moving in a forward direction. These are the 27th acupressure points on the kidney meridian and located directly beneath the clavicle bones.

2 Place either hand (or both) at the bottom of the trunk of your body and then slide your hand up the center.

3 Take a deep breath in as you move your hands slowly straight up the center of your body, to your lower lip.

4 Continue upward, bringing your hands past your lips and exuberantly raising them into the sky. Exhale. Circle your arms back to your pelvis and repeat 3 times.

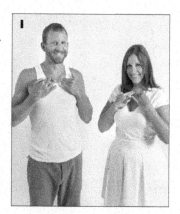

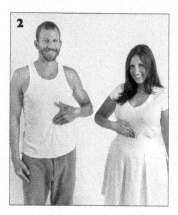

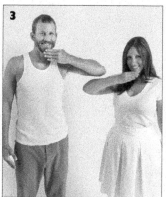

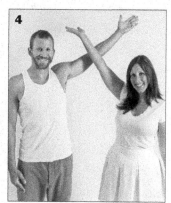

The

FIVE-MINUTE DAILY

ENERGY ROUTINE

What the Five-Minute Daily Energy Routine Is and How It Works

We are now going to combine several of the techniques into a five-minute routine. The Five-Minute Daily Energy Routine is like pressing a reset button, helping restore your body's natural energy flows. This routine will strengthen your immune system, making you less vulnerable and more resilient, as it:

- Provides a general energy balancing
- Helps restore your vitality
- Grounds you and stabilizes your force fields
- Helps you feel better instantly
- Develops positive habits in your energy system

After working with more than ten thousand clients in 90-minute individual sessions, giving most of them back-home assignments and watching what occurred, I found that these techniques are the most potent and have the most positive impact for just about everyone. They help your body not only to come into balance but to be more protected from environmental radiation, pollutants, and toxins.

I know it is no small thing to suggest that you build another routine into your life. We are all extraordinarily busy, an epidemic of modern life. But some investments pay off. I promise you that the Daily Energy Routine, practiced regularly, will give you a good return, in terms of how you feel and function, on the small daily investment it requires.

I know from experience that you will be more likely to maintain a program like this if you tie it into an activity you already do. If you exercise regularly, or do yoga, tai chi, or Pilates, it can be a great warm-up or cooldown. If you meditate, it can bring you into a centered space from which you can go deeper. Some people, particularly those who are not morning persons, do it before they get out of bed. Some people do it as a kind of transition ritual when they get home from work. Some people do it as part of their bath or shower. It doesn't matter in which order you do the exercises, and the more comfortable you are, the better.

The Five-Minute Daily Energy
Routine Exercises

THE ZIP-UP

Briskly tap the K-27 points to assure that your meridians are moving in a forward direction. These are the 27th acupressure points on the kidney meridian and located directly beneath the clavicle bones. Place your hands at the bottom of the trunk of your body and then slide your hand up the center. Take a deep breath in as you move your hands slowly straight up the center of your body, to your lower lip. Continue upward, bringing your hands past your lips and exuberantly raising them into the sky. Exhale. Circle your arms back to your pelvis and repeat 3 times.

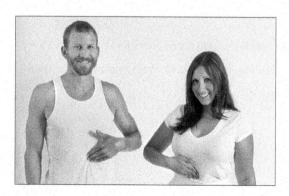

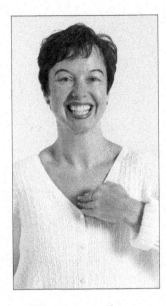

The thymus thump

THE FOUR THUMPS

1 *Place the pads of your fingers beneath your cheekbones, next to your nose. Thump firmly for 15 seconds. This helps to drain sinuses and clear the lymph glands in the neck. It can also release tension and reduce excessive worry.*

2 *Place your forefingers on your collarbone and move them inward toward the U-shaped notch at the top of your breastbone (about where a man would tie his tie). Move your fingers to the bottom of the U. Then go to the left and right about an inch and thump firmly for 10 to 15 seconds.*

3 *Place the fingers of either or both hands in the center of your sternum, at the thymus gland. Thump firmly for about 10 to 15 seconds.*

4 *Thump the neurolymphatic spleen points firmly for 10 to 15 seconds with your fingers or knuckles. They are beneath the breasts and down one rib.*

THE HOMOLATERAL/CROSS-CRAWL EXERCISE

While standing, lift your left arm and left leg simultaneously. As you let them down, raise your right arm and right leg. Repeat several times. Lift your left arm and right leg simultaneously. As you let them down, raise your right arm and left leg. Repeat several times.

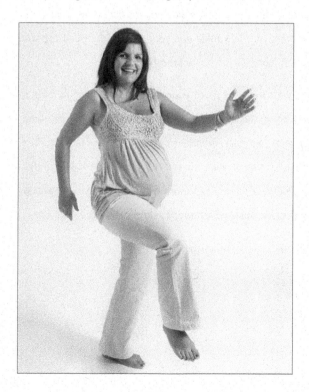

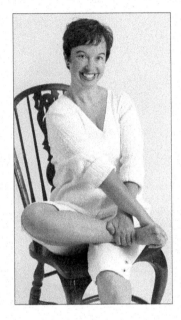

WAYNE COOK POSTURE

1 Place your right foot over your left knee. Wrap your left hand around your right ankle and your right hand around the ball of your right foot. Breathe in slowly through your nose and out through your mouth. Repeat this 4 to 5 times. Switch to the other foot. Place your left foot over your right knee. Wrap your right hand around your left ankle and your left hand around the ball of your left foot. Use the same breathing.

2 Uncross your legs and place your fingertips together forming a pyramid. Bring your thumbs to rest on your "third eye" just above the bridge of your nose. Breathe slowly in through your nose. Then breathe out through your mouth, repeating this 4 or 5 times. Finally, allow your thumbs to separate slowly across your forehead, pulling the skin. Allow your hands to simply drop into your lap.

THE CROWN PULL

1 Apply pressure to forehead and slowly pull your fingers apart, stretching the skin. Breathe deeply, in through your nose and out through your mouth. Next, place your fingertips on the top of your head and repeat the stretch.

2 Repeat this pattern starting at the top, center, and back of your head. Continue until you reach the base of your neck.

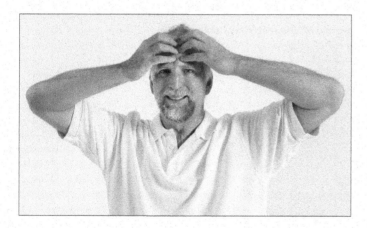

THE SPINAL FLUSH

Lean into a chair or wall, or lie facedown. Partner should deeply massage on either side of the spine, from the base of the neck to the bottom of the sacrum. The thumbs are used to apply deep pressure in a circular motion for about 5 seconds on each point. Once at the bottom of your sacrum, your partner can repeat the spinal flush or "sweep" the energies off the body. From the shoulder, and with an open hand, your partner sweeps all the way down the back, down the legs, and off the feet, 2 or 3 times.

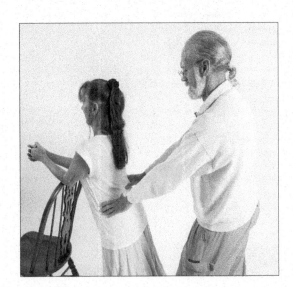

THE HOOKUP

Place one hand with your middle finger in your navel and the other hand with your middle finger in your "third eye" (between your eyebrows). Push in and pull up.

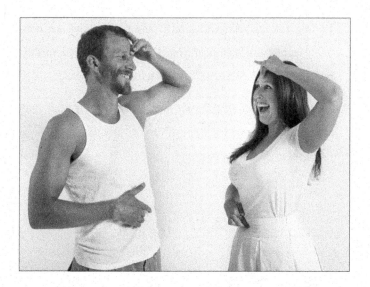

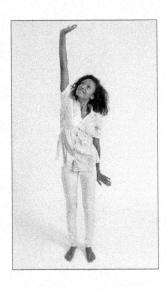

CONNECTING HEAVEN AND EARTH

1 *Start with your hands on your thighs, with your fingers spread.*

2 *Inhale through your nose, bring your arms out and together in a prayer position. Exhale through your mouth.*

3 *Inhaling through your nose, stretch one arm up and one arm down, pushing with your palms. Hold, exhale through your mouth, and return to the prayer position. Switch arms and repeat.*

4 *Drop your arms down, fold your body forward at the waist, and relax with your knees slightly bent. Take two breaths before slowly returning to a standing position.*

FOR ADDITIONAL STUDY

1. *Energy Medicine* (book and DVDs)
2. *Energy Medicine for Women* (book and DVDs)
3. *Promise of Energy Psychology* (book and DVDs)
4. Classes and workshops, www.innersource.net and www.DondiDahlin.com
5. www.LearnEnergyMedicine.com

ABOUT THE AUTHORS

DONNA EDEN

For more than three decades, Donna Eden has been teaching people how to work with the body's energy systems to reclaim their health and natural vitality.

Donna is among the world's most sought, most joyous, and most authoritative spokespersons for Energy Medicine. Her abilities as a healer are legendary. She has taught some eighty thousand people worldwide, both laypeople and professionals, how to understand the body as an energy system.

Able from childhood to clairvoyantly see the body's subtle energies, she not only works with those energies to further health, happiness, and vitality, she has made a career of teaching people who do not see subtle energies how to work with them—joyfully and effectively.

Donna has taught hundreds of self-empowering, alternative health workshops throughout the world that have been attended by more than eighty thousand participants. Her first book, *Energy Medicine*, is the classic in its field, with more than 200,000 sales.

It has been translated into fifteen languages and has won two national book awards. Its sequel, *Energy Medicine for Women*, received the "best health book" award in the prestigious Nautilus competition.

As a healer, Donna Eden has treated over ten thousand individual clients. She is widely referenced in the alternative health field, and many of her workshop attendees include physicians, nurses, and other mainstream health professionals. Donna consistently exhilarates and amazes her audiences. Her work is available in books, on DVD, and in live training programs. See www.LearnEnergyMedicine.com.

"The contribution Donna Eden has made with Energy Medicine will stand as one of the backbone studies as we lay a sound foundation for the field of holistic medicine."

—CAROLINE MYSS, PH.D.

DONDI DAHLIN

Dondi, Donna's younger daughter, was raised with Energy Medicine as an everyday part of her life. Dondi has continued to use Energy Medicine in her careers as a successful actress and professional dancer who has toured the world, teaching and performing in more than twenty countries. She has won many dance, speaking, and drama awards, is a member of the Screen Actors Guild, and has published several articles about Middle Eastern dance and her life in the Middle East. Dondi is now a mom and teaching her son, Tiernan Ray, the beauty, magic, and importance of Energy Medicine. See www.DondiDahlin.com.

MODEL CREDITS

Rick Cabados

Dondi Dahlin

Titanya Dahlin

Albert Devenyns

Monique Devenyns

Roger Devenyns

Anna Valencia Goebel

Michelle Grangetto

Steve Grangetto

Jacob Grosz

Christopher W. Jones

Jiana Jordan

Terry Lamb

Uriah Lamb

Cassie Mavis

Magdalena Montrond

Mariela Shibley

Ben Singer

Lindsay Southall

Rick Unis

Bernadette Unis-Johnston

Sabina Wong

INDEX

toxic, 20 (see *also* Toxins,
environmental)
Exhaustion, 29, 56
See also Fatigue
Expelling the Venom, 26–27

F
Fatigue, 6, 34
See also Exhaustion
Fear
irrational, 28
reducing, 29, 41, 54
Fear Tap, 28–29
Fight-or-flight response,
40, 41
Five-Minute Daily Energy Routine,
61–64
exercises comprising, 20, 24, 32, 44,
48, 56, 58, 65–71, 72
Flow, 3, 4
of energy. *See* Meridians of
information between brain
hemispheres, 42
Flowing energy, 1
Flu, 9
Fluorescent lights, 17
Focus, mental, 8, 22, 50
Food, metabolism of, 32
Food and Drug Administration
(FDA), 7
Force fields, bioenergetic, 22, 56
stabilizing, 63
Forebrain, 38, 40–41
Four Memory Pumps, 30–31
Four Thumps, 32–33
Frustration, 26, 27
Fuzzy thinking, 42

G
Gait Reflexes, 34–35
Gallbladder meridian, 11
Governing meridian, 44, 46

H
Habits
for managing stress, 54
positive, 63
unwanted, repatterning, 40
Happiness, 1, 8, 20
creating patterns of, 52
See also Joy
Harmony, 3, 4, 12
Headaches, 5, 9
alleviating, 24
Healing, 36–37
ancient traditions, 3, 12, 28
interference of medications with, 7
self-, 6, 7
speeding, 42
Healing Touch, 4
Health insurance, 9
Heart, 16, 28
Heart chakra, 36, 37
Heaven Rushing In, 36–37
High blood pressure, 5, 9, 50
High-voltage wires, 17
Hip pain, 36
Holding Another's Stress Points,
38–39
Holding Your Own Stress Points,
40–41
Holistic medicine, 76
Homolateral March, 43
Homolateral/Cross-Crawl
Repatterning, 42–43

Metabolism, 11, 32
Mood swings, 5
Muscular system, 12

N

Negative energy, 58
Neolithic period, 3
Nervous system, 30, 45
   autonomic, 55
   calming, 24
   central, 53, 58
   resetting, 42
   tapping into, 52
Neurolymphatic reflex points, 49
Neurolymphatic spleen points, 33, 66
Neurotransmitters, 33
Neurovascular points, 38, 40, 41

O

Oxygen, 20, 30
Oz, Dr., 4

P

Pain, 5–7
   emotional, 13
   physical, 13, 36
Panic, 50, 51
Pathways, energy, 3, 11, 58
   See also Meridians
Performance, 22, 56
   peak, 4
Pharmaceutical companies, 6
Pilates, 64
Pills. See Drugs
Pollutants, 64
   energy, 17
Positive thinking, 52, 58

Postures, 3
   See also Wayne Cook Posture
Preventive medicine, 9
Psychological problems, 5

Q

Qi gong, 3

R

Radiation, environmental, 64
Rage, 26
   See also Anger
Reiki, 4
Relaxation techniques, 13, 34, 38
Renewal, feelings of, 3
Respiratory system, 12
Righteous anger, 26
Running, 16

S

Scared, feeling. See Fear
Sedentary lifestyles, 16
Seizures, 45, 56
Self-care, 4
Sensitivity, emotional, 55
Sex life, improving, 13
Shiatsu, 3
Shock, 55
Short-term memory, restoring, 30
Sinuses, draining, 32, 66
Skeletal system, 12
Sleep disturbance, 4
   See also Insomnia
Spinal Flush, 48–49
Spirituality, 24, 36
Spleen meridian, 10
Spleen points, neurolymphatic, 33, 66